Contents

What is the Autoimmune Protocol Diet?

The Autoimmune Protocol (AIP) is a diet that aims to reduce inflammation, pain, and other symptoms caused by autoimmune diseases, such as lupus, inflammatory bowel disease (IBD), celiac disease, and rheumatoid arthritis

A healthy immune system is designed to produce antibodies that attack foreign or harmful cells in your body.

However, in people with autoimmune disorders, the immune system tends to produce antibodies that, rather than fight infections, attack healthy cells and tissues.

This can result in a range of symptoms, including joint pain, fatigue, abdominal pain, diarrhea, brain fog, and tissue and nerve damage.

A few examples of autoimmune disorders include rheumatoid arthritis, lupus, IBD, type 1 diabetes, and psoriasis.

Autoimmune diseases are thought to be caused by a variety of factors, including genetic propensity, infection, stress, inflammation, and medication use.

Also, some research suggests that, in susceptible individuals, damage to the gut barrier can lead to increased intestinal permeability, also known as "leaky gut," which may trigger the development of certain autoimmune diseases

Certain foods are believed to possibly increase the gut's permeability, thereby increasing your likelihood of leaky gut.

The AIP diet focuses on eliminating these foods and replacing them with health-promoting, nutrient-dense foods that are thought to help heal the gut, and ultimately, reduce inflammation and symptoms of autoimmune diseases.

It also removes certain ingredients like gluten, which may cause abnormal immune responses in susceptible individuals.

While experts believe that a leaky gut may be a plausible explanation for the inflammation experienced by people with autoimmune disorders, they warn that the current research makes it impossible to confirm a cause-and-effect relationship between the two.

Therefore, more research is needed before strong conclusions can be made.

How does it work?

The AIP diet resembles the paleo diet, both in the types of foods allowed and avoided, as well as in the phases that comprise it. Due to their similarities, many consider the AIP diet an extension of the paleo diet — though AIP may be seen as a stricter version of it.

The AIP diet consists of two main phases.

The elimination phase

The first phase is an elimination phase that involves the removal of foods and medications believed to cause gut inflammation, imbalances between levels of good and bad bacteria in the gut, or an immune response.

During this phase, foods like grains, legumes, nuts, seeds, nightshade vegetables, eggs, and dairy are completely avoided.

Tobacco, alcohol, coffee, oils, food additives, refined and processed sugars, and certain medications, such as non-steroidal anti-inflammatory drugs (NSAIDs) should also be avoided.

Examples of NSAIDs include ibuprofen, naproxen, diclofenac, and high dose aspirin.

On the other hand, this phase encourages the consumption of fresh, nutrient-dense foods, minimally processed meat, fermented foods, and bone broth. It also emphasizes the improvement of lifestyle factors, such as stress, sleep, and physical activity.

The length of the elimination phase of the diet varies, as it's typically maintained until a person feels a noticeable reduction in symptoms. On average, most people maintain this phase for 30–90 days, but some may notice improvements as early as within the first 3 weeks.

The reintroduction phase

Once a measurable improvement in symptoms and overall well-being occurs, the reintroduction phase can begin. During this phase, the avoided foods are gradually reintroduced into the diet, one at a time, based on the person's tolerance.

The goal of this phase is to identify which foods contribute to a person's symptoms and reintroduce all foods that don't cause any symptoms while continuing to avoid those that do. This allows for the widest dietary variety a person can tolerate.

During this phase, foods should be reintroduced one at a time, allowing for a period of 5–7 days before reintroducing a different food. This allows a person enough time to notice if any of their symptoms reappear before continuing the reintroduction process.

Foods that are well tolerated can be added back into the diet, while those that trigger symptoms should continue to be avoided. Keep in mind that your food tolerance may change over time.

As such, you may want to repeat the reintroduction test for foods that initially failed the test every once in a while.

Step-by-step reintroduction protocol

Here's a step-by-step approach to reintroducing foods that were avoided during the elimination phase of the AIP diet.

• Step 1. Choose one food to reintroduce. Plan to consume this food a few times per day on the testing day, then avoid it completely for 5–6 days.

• Step 2. Eat a small amount, such as 1 teaspoon of the food, and wait 15 minutes to see if you have a reaction.

• Step 3. If you experience any symptoms, end the test and avoid this food. If you have no symptoms, eat a slightly larger portion, such as 1 1/2 tablespoons, of the same food and monitor how you feel for 2–3 hours.

• Step 4. If you experience any symptoms over this period, end the test and avoid this food. If no symptoms occur, eat a normal portion of the same food and avoid it for 5–6 days without reintroducing any other foods.

• Step 5. If you experience no symptoms for 5–6 days, you may reincorporate the tested food into your diet, and repeat this 5-step reintroduction process with a new food.

It's best to avoid reintroducing foods under circumstances that tend to increase inflammation and make it difficult to interpret results. These include during an infection, following a poor night's sleep, when feeling unusually stressed, or following a strenuous workout.

Additionally, it's sometimes recommended to reintroduce foods in a particular order. For example, when reintroducing dairy, choose dairy products with the lowest lactose concentration to reintroduce first, such as ghee or fermented dairy products.

Foods to eat and avoid

The AIP diet has strict recommendations regarding which foods to eat or avoid during its elimination phase.

Foods to avoid

- Grains: rice, wheat, oats, barley, rye, etc., as well as foods derived from them, such as pasta, bread, and breakfast cereals

- Legumes: lentils, beans, peas, peanuts, etc., as well as foods derived from them, such as tofu, tempeh, mock meats, or peanut butter

- Nightshade vegetables: eggplants, peppers, potatoes, tomatoes, tomatillos, etc., as well as spices derived from nightshade vegetables, such as paprika

- Eggs: whole eggs, egg whites, or foods containing these ingredients

- Dairy: cow's, goat's, or sheep's milk, as well as foods derived from these milks, such as cream, cheese, butter, or ghee; dairy-based protein powders or other supplements should also be avoided

• Nuts and seeds: all nuts and seeds and foods derived from them, such as flours, butter, or oils; also includes cocoa and seed-based spices, such as coriander, cumin, anise, fennel, fenugreek, mustard, and nutmeg

• Certain beverages: alcohol and coffee

• Processed vegetable oils: canola, rapeseed, corn, cottonseed, palm kernel, safflower, soybean, or sunflower oils

• Refined or processed sugars: cane or beet sugar, corn syrup, brown rice syrup, and barley malt syrup; also includes sweets, soda, candy, frozen desserts, and chocolate, which may contain these ingredients

- Food additives and artificial sweeteners: trans fats, food colorings, emulsifiers, and thickeners, as well as artificial sweeteners, such as stevia, mannitol, and xylitol

Some AIP protocols further recommend avoiding all fruit — both fresh or dried — during the elimination phase. Others allow the inclusion of 10–40 grams of fructose per day, which amounts to around 1–2 portions of fruit per day.

Although not specified in all AIP protocols, some also suggest avoiding algae, such as spirulina or chlorella, during the elimination phase, as this type of sea vegetable may also stimulate an immune response.

Foods to eat

- Vegetables: a variety of vegetables except for nightshade vegetables and algae, which should be avoided

- Fresh fruit: a variety of fresh fruit, in moderation

- Tubers: sweet potatoes, taro, yams, as well as Jerusalem or Chinese artichokes

- Minimally processed meat: wild game, fish, seafood, organ meat, and poultry; meats should be wild, grass-fed or pasture-raised, whenever possible

- Fermented, probiotic-rich foods: nondairy-based fermented food, such as kombucha, kimchi, sauerkraut, pickles, and coconut kefir; probiotic supplements may also be consumed

- Minimally processed vegetable oils: olive oil, avocado oil, or coconut oil

- Herbs and spices: as long as they're not derived from a seed

- Vinegars: balsamic, apple cider, and red wine vinegar, as long as they're free of added sugars

- Natural sweeteners: maple syrup and honey, in moderation

- Certain teas: green and black tea at average intakes of up to 3–4 cups per day

- Bone broth

Despite being allowed, some protocols further recommend that you moderate your intake of salt, saturated and omega-6 fats, natural sugars, such as honey or maple syrup, as well as coconut-based foods.

Depending on the AIP protocol at hand, small amounts of fruit may also be allowed. This usually amounts to a maximum intake of 10–40 grams of fructose per day, or the equivalent of about 1–2 portions of fresh fruit.

Some protocols further suggest moderating your intake of high glycemic fruits and vegetables, including dried fruit, sweet potatoes, and plantain.

The glycemic index (GI) is a system used to rank foods on a scale of 0 to 100, based on how much they will increase blood sugar levels, compared with white bread. High glycemic fruits and vegetables are those ranked 70 or above on the GI scale.

Does the AIP diet work?

Though research on the AIP diet is limited, some evidence suggests that it may reduce inflammation and symptoms of certain autoimmune diseases.

May help heal a leaky gut

People with autoimmune diseases often have a leaky gut, and experts believe there may be a link between the inflammation they experience and the permeability of their gut.

A healthy gut typically has a low permeability. This allows it to act as a good barrier and prevent food and waste remains from leaking into the bloodstream.

However, a highly permeable or leaky gut allows foreign particles to crossover into the bloodstream, in turn, possibly causing inflammation.

In parallel, there's growing evidence that the foods you eat can influence your gut's immunity and function, and in some cases, possibly even reduce the degree of inflammation you experience.

One hypothesis entertained by researchers is that by helping heal leaky gut, the AIP diet may help reduce the degree of inflammation a person experiences.

Although scientific evidence is currently limited, a handful of studies suggests that the AIP diet may help reduce inflammation or symptoms caused by it, at least among a subset of people with certain autoimmune disorders.

However, more research is needed to specifically understand the exact ways in which the AIP diet may help, as well as the precise circumstances under which it may do so.

May reduce inflammation and symptoms of some autoimmune disorders

To date, the AIP diet has been tested in a small group of people and yielded seemingly positive results.

For instance, in a recent 11-week study in 15 people with IBD on an AIP diet, participants reported experiencing significantly fewer IBD-related symptoms by the end of the study. However, no significant changes in markers of inflammation were observed.

Similarly, a small study had people with IBD follow the AIP diet for 11 weeks. Participants reported significant improvements in bowel frequency, stress, and the ability to perform leisure or sport activities as early as 3 weeks into the study.

In another study, 16 women with Hashimoto's thyroiditis, an autoimmune disorder affecting the thyroid gland, followed the AIP diet for 10 weeks. By the end of the study, inflammation and disease-related symptoms decreased by 29% and 68%, respectively.

Participants also reported significant improvements in their quality of life, despite there being no significant differences in their measures of thyroid function.

Although promising, studies remain small and few. Also, to date, they have only been performed on a small subset of people with autoimmune disorders. Therefore, more research is needed before strong conclusions can be made.

Should you try it?

The AIP diet is designed to help reduce inflammation, pain, or other symptoms caused by autoimmune diseases. As such, it may work best for people with autoimmune diseases, such as lupus, IBD, celiac disease, or rheumatoid arthritis.

Autoimmune diseases cannot be cured, but their symptoms may be managed. The AIP diet aims to help you do so by helping you identify which foods may be triggering your specific symptoms.

Evidence regarding the efficacy of this diet is currently limited to people with IBD and Hashimoto's disease.

However, based on the way in which this diet is believed to function, people with other autoimmune diseases may benefit from it, too.

There are currently few downsides to giving this diet a try, especially when performed under the supervision of a dietitian or other medical professional.

Seeking professional guidance prior to giving the AIP diet a try will help you better pinpoint which foods may be causing your specific symptoms, as well as ensure that you continue to meet your nutrient requirements as best as possible throughout all phases of this diet.

EASY 7-DAY AIP DIET MEAL PLAN

Just because AIP is super restrictive doesn't mean you can't eat well. We've made an easy 7-day meal plan for you that's specifically based on the elimination phase.

Day 1

- Breakfast: Fruit salad with bananas, strawberries, and blueberries

- Lunch: Oven-baked salmon with lemon slices over a bed of arugula

- Snack: Fresh cucumber

- Dinner: Ground beef patties

Day 2

- Breakfast: Sweet potato hash with steak

- Lunch: Turkey breast and avocado

- Snack: Chomps sea salt beef jerky stick

- Dinner: Chicken thighs and asparagus

Day 3

- Breakfast: Sautéed ham and spinach.

- Lunch: Kale chips and chicken breast.

- Snack: A can of tuna

• Dinner: Bunless mushroom burger

Day 4

• Breakfast: Mushroom and onion mix with pork loin

• Lunch: Creamy AIP chicken salad

• Snack: Pickles

• Dinner: Roasted squash, broccoli, and grilled tilapia

Day 5

• Breakfast: Chicken livers and spinach

• Lunch: Turkey burgers

• Snack: Chomps italian style beef jerky stick

• Dinner: Roasted duck and brussel sprouts

Day 6

- Breakfast: AIP porridge

- Lunch: Sweet potato chicken poppers

- Snack: Fresh melon and honey

- Dinner: Shrimp over zucchini pasta

Day 7

- Breakfast: Blueberry coconut smoothie

- Lunch: Grilled chicken tenders and asparagus

- Snack: Dried fruit

- Dinner: Coconut shrimp and grits

ADDITIONAL AIP SNACK OPTIONS

Many of us rely on carb-loaded foods like bread to help us stay full, and we don't realize how much we rely on them until we stop eating them.

Here are a few more common AIP snacks to help get you through those hunger pangs:

- AIP granola

- Avocados

- Tuna

- Berries

- Cucumbers

- Root vegetable fries

- Pemmican

- Pickles

- AIP trail mix

- Chomps beef sticks

Autoimmune Diet Recipes

You may not be able to eat all the foods you're used to, but you're still in for a delicious meal plan. Avocado, coconut milk, ghee, and grass-fed meat make this a diet rich in healthy fats, and you'll also get plenty of other nutrient-dense foods like leafy green vegetables, sweet potatoes, squashes, berries, and more.

Instant Pot Beef Stock

Preparation time

2 hours 15 minutes

Ingredients

- 3-4 lb Beef bones, grass-fed, roasted

- 3 whole Carrots, cut in half

- 4 whole Celery, ribs

- 1 Onion, sliced in half

- 2 cloves Garlic, smashed with a knive

- 1 Bay Leaf

- 1 tsp Himalayan Pink Salt

- 1 Tbsp Apple Cider Vinegar

- 1 Instant Pot

Instructions

1. Preheat your oven to bake at 420 degrees.

2. Place the beef bones in a glass baking sheet, and sprinkle with salt if desired.

3. Roast the bones for 30 minutes, flip them to their other side, and then roast for another 20 minutes.

4. While the bones are roasting, prepare the vegetables for the broth.

5. Place the roasted bones into your Instant Pot, and then add the carrot, celery, onion, garlic, bay leaf, salt, and apple cider vinegar.

6. Fill the Instant Pot with filtered water until it reaches about an inch below the max fill line.

7. Place the lid on, and seal, and set to manual high pressure for 75 minutes.

8. Once the broth is finished, remove the large bones and vegetable pieces, and then strain the broth through a fine mesh strainer.

9. Pour the strained broth back into the Instant Pot, if using immediately after for soup, or allow to cool and freeze for future use.

Autoimmune-Friendly Apple Pie

Preparation time

2 minutes

Ingredients

- 5 whole Apple, Granny Smith, peeled, quartered, cored, and sliced thinly

- 1/2 cup Coconut Palm Sugar, + 2 Tbsp

- 1 Tbsp Cinnamon, ground

- 1/4 tsp Sea Salt, + 1/4 tsp

- 1 whole Lemon, juiced

- 1 cup Arrowroot Flour

- 1/2 cup Coconut Flour

- 3/4 cup Coconut Oil, Organic, cold

- 1/2 cup Water, cold

Instructions

1. Preheat your oven to 350 degrees. If you haven't measured out your coconut oil and water and then placed them in the refrigerator to cool, do it now.

2. Place the apple slices in a large bowl. Fill a large pot with enough water to soak all of the apple slices, and bring it to a boil. When it is hot, pour the water into the bowl with the apples until they are just covered. Let them sit in the hot water for 8 minutes, and then place in a colander to drain and set aside while you make the crust.

3. To make the crust, combine the arrowroot, coconut flour, palm sugar, and sea salt in a medium bowl and stir to combine. Using a pastry cutter, butterknives, or your fingers, cut in the cold coconut oil until you have pea-sized lumps. Add the cold water, and mix gently. The mixture will be crumbly and not like regular dough--don't over mix!

4. Place the mixture into a 9-inch pie dish. Using your fingers, spread it evenly across the bottoms and up the sides. Prick some holes in the bottom of the crust with a fork. Again, the dough will not behave like regular pie dough, and the less you handle it the more flaky it will come out. Bake for 15 minutes and then set aside while you make the filling.

5. Lay out a clean kitchen towel and pour the apple slices on it, blotting them dry. Combine the coconut palm sugar, cinnamon, and salt in a large bowl, and then add the dry apple slices and mix gently. Pour the mixture into the crust, arranging the slices as needed.Sprinkle the pie with lemon juice and place in the oven to cook for 30-35 minutes, until the crust is golden brown.

6. Let cool for 10-15 minutes and then serve.

Roasted Chicken Thighs

Preparation time

1 hour 15 minutes

Ingredients

- 1 tsp Avocado Oil

- 12 cloves Garlic, (a fist, unpeeled)

- 4 Chicken Thigh, skin on

- 1 tsp Primal Palate Super Gyro Seasoning

- pinch Himalayan Pink Salt

Instructions

1. Preheat your oven to 350 F.

2. Heat a medium pot over medium heat with the avocado oil, and saute the garlic cloves for 2-3 minutes (until the skins begin to brown.

3. In a large skillet over medium high heat, sear the chicken thighs on both sides (do skin-side first so they do not stick) - about 2-3 minutes per side.

4. Place the chicken over the garlic, and season with salt and Primal Palate Super Gyro blend.

5. Bake for an hour, covered. Serve along side your choice of vegetable.

Roasted Chicken & Veggies

Preparation time

1 hour 30 minutes

Ingredients

- 1 lb Sweet Potato, frozen and cubed, or sub another starchy vegetable

- 2 Tbsp Olive Oil, Extra Virgin, divided

- 7/8 tsp Salt, divided

- 2 3/4 tsp Primal Palate Garlic & Herb Seasoning, divided, or sub your favorite seasoning blend

- 1 lb Broccoli, florets, or sub other vegetable

- 3 1/2 lb Chicken, Whole

Instructions

1. Preheat oven to 425°F.

2. Toss sweet potatoes in 1 Tbsp olive oil with about 1/4 tsp salt and 1/2 tsp seasoning blend (or just season to taste!).

3. Place in the bottom of a roasting pan.

4. Season the broccoli with about 1/8 tsp salt and 1/4 tsp of the seasoning blend (once again, you can just season to taste if you like).

5. Add this to the roasting pan with the sweet potatoes.

6. Rinse the chicken, if desired, and pat dry with a paper towel.

7.   Rub the skin with 1 Tbsp olive oil and about 1/2 tsp salt and 2 tsp seasoning blend.

8. Secure the legs and wings to the chicken with kitchen twine and place in the middle of the roasting dish.

9.   Breast-up, breast-down... I know everyone argues about that so I'll leave it up to you. I did mine breast-up so if you do-breast down, it may cook differently. You may want to scoot the vegetables out from under the chicken to around the edges of the pan.

10. Cover the roasting pan with foil and bake for 45 minutes. This prevents the spices from burning.

11. After 45 minutes, remove the foil and continue baking until the temperature of the

chicken reaches 165°F. You can check for doneness by inserting a meat thermometer into the meatiest part of the inner thigh but make sure it's not touching bone. It will likely take another 20-30 minutes to fully cook after removing the foil.

Delicata Squash Super Gyro Sliders

Preparation time

50 minutes

Ingredients

- 2 lb Ground Beef, grass fed, 85% lean

- 2 whole Delicata Squash

- 1 Tbsp Primal Palate Super Gyro Seasoning

- 5 pieces Bacon

- 1 whole Avocado

- 4 sprig Cilantro

- 1 whole Lime

- 1/2 tsp Himalayan Pink Salt

Instructions

1. Pre-heat oven to 400F.

2. Place your bacon strips flat on the sheet pan and place in the cold oven while it pre-heats.

3. Cook bacon here for 10-15 minutes, until crispy.

4. Remove from the oven when done to your liking. Do not turn oven off.

5. Drain some of the fat off the sheet pan into a ramekin, set aside.

6. Leave about 2 tbsp on the sheet pan.

7. Slice your delicate squash into 1/2 inch rings.

8. Use a spoon to remove the seeds.

9. Place your rings on the greased sheet pan and flip over to grease both sides of the rings with bacon fat.

10. Sprinkle lightly with salt, about 1/4 tsp, save the rest.

11. Place the squash in the oven.

12. Bake for 15 minutes. Then gently flip the rings over.

13. Bake another 5 minutes, or until fork tender.

14. In the meantime, in a large bowl mix the ground beef, seasoning, salt and bacon fat. Shape 6-8 sliders.

15. Remove the squash from the oven.

16. Use a spatula to remove the squash from the sheet pan, set aside.

17. Arrange burger sliders on the sheet pan and roast at 400F for 15 minutes.

18. When they are done, place a slider over each ring.

19. Peel your avocado and smash it.

20. Spoon a littler over each patty.

21. Sprinkle a little salt over them, then a little lime juice.

22. Top with a few cilantro leaves.

23. Lastly, cut up the bacon in to 1/2 inch chunks and top your sliders off.

24. Viola! Delectable, seasonal, satisfying!

Anti-Inflammatory Turmeric Tea

Preparation time

12 minutes

Ingredients

- 1 cup Water

- 1/4 tsp Turmeric Powder

- 1/4 tsp Cinnamon, ground

- 1/4 tsp Ginger, ground

- 1/2 tsp Honey, Raw

- 1 Tbsp Lemon Juice

- Buy on Amazon

Instructions

1. In a small saucepan, bring the water to a steam (not quite to a boil, the hotter it gets, the longer you have to wait for it to cool.)

2. Add the spices, honey and lemon juice, and stir to combine.

3. Remove the saucepan from heat, and cover with a lid.

4. Allow the mixture to steam and combine for 10 minutes.

5. Drink once cooled.

Note

1. This tea will settle as you drink it, so you will need a spoon to redistribute the spices.

Mashed Cauliflower

Preparation time

30 minutes

Ingredients

- 1 whole Cauliflower

- 1 1/2 cup Baby Bella Mushrooms, or one 6 oz package

- 4 cup Arugula

- 6 pieces Bacon

- 1/4 cup Coconut Milk, you'll add this 1 Tbsp at a time, and may not use it all

- 3 Tbsp Coconut Aminos

- 1 Tbsp Unflavored Gelatin, Beef, Great Lakes brand

- 1 Tbsp Nutritional Yeast

- 2 Tbsp Bacon Grease, I suggest reserving grease from cooking the bacon, but you can also use ghee, coconut oil, or avocado oil

- 1 Tbsp Olive Oil, Extra Virgin

- 2 tsp Sea Salt, or season to taste

Instructions

FOR THE MASHED CAULIFLOWER

1. Start by removing the leafy part of the stem, and roughly chop the head of cauliflower. It's

okay to include the rest of the stem since the cauliflower will be steamed and blended.

2. Steam chopped cauliflower using your method of choice. I recommend a stovetop method.

3. Add steamed cauliflower to a blender or food processor. You can also do this with an immersion blender or by hand, but I find the blender and food processor to be the simplest and tends to yield the best consistency.

4. Add nutritional yeast (optional to provide a cheesy flavor), gelatin (to provide a thicker texture), about 1-2 tsp sea salt, and 1 Tbsp coconut milk. You'll want to start with just 1 Tbsp coconut milk, but you'll likely need more depending on how much moisture is retained in your cauliflower.

5. Blend until smooth. Increase coconut milk by the tablespoon until desired consistency is reached. Be sure to test cauliflower to make sure it's salted to your liking.

FOR THE MUSHROOMS

1. Heat oil in a sauté pan over medium low heat.

2. Slice mushrooms in half and add to sauté pan. Cook slowly over low heat for the flavors to fully develop.

3. When the mushrooms are well cooked, pour in the Coconut Aminos to deglaze the pan and develop a caramelization on the outside of the mushrooms.

4. Remove from heat and sprinkle with a bit of coarse sea salt while the glaze is still wet.

FOR THE BACON

1. Preheat oven to 375 degrees.

2. Lay bacon on a rimmed, parchment lined baking sheet. Cook until crisp, about 12-15 minutes.

3. Remove bacon from cooking sheet and set aside to cool on a paper towel. This will absorb extra grease. Reserve the grease left on the baking sheet and store in an airtight jar in the fridge to use for cooking.

4. Once bacon has cooled, rough chop and store until use.

ASSEMBLY

1. Divide ingredients among 2 bowls, and drizzle with olive or avocado oil. Sprinkle with coarse sea salt.

2. These ingredients can be prepped the day before and reheated for a quick breakfast bowl, or eaten straight from the fridge.

AIP Banana Mug Cake

Preparation time

5 minutes

Ingredients

- 1 whole Banana, peeled

- 1 Tbsp Coconut Oil, Organic, solid, not melted

- 2 Tbsp Coconut Milk

- 1/2 tsp Pure Vanilla Extract

- 2 Tbsp Coconut Flour

- 1 tsp Cinnamon, ground

- 1/4 tsp Baking Soda

Instructions

1. Mash the banana and add the coconut oil, coconut milk, and vanilla.

2. Add the coconut flour, cinnamon, and baking soda; mix well.

3. Transfer to a ramekin or coffee cup.

4. Microwave on HIGH (100 percent power) for 3 minutes.

5. Cool a bit and enjoy.

Autoimmune-Friendly Pumpkin Spice Cake w/ Gingersnap Crust

Preparation time

1 hour

Ingredients

- 3/4 cup Arrowroot Powder, + 1/3 cup

- 1/4 tsp Sea Salt, + 1/4 tsp

- 1 1/2 cups Dates (Medjool), pitted and soaked in hot water for 5 minutes

- 1 1/2 tsp Ginger Root, grated

- 3 cups Pumpkin Puree

- 1/2 cup Maple Syrup, Pure, + 2 tbsp

- 1/4 cup Lard, (or coconut oil), + 2.5 Tbsp, + 2 Tbsp

- 2 1/2 Tbsp Unflavored Gelatin, Beef, Great Lakes brand

- 1 1/2 tsp Cinnamon, ground

- 1/4 tsp Cloves, ground

- 2 Tbsp Honey, Raw

Instructions

1. Preheat the oven to 325 degrees F and grease an 8- inch spring-form pan with either lard or coconut oil.

2. Drain the dates, and place all of the ingredients in a food processor and process for a minute, until a thick and sticky mixture forms. You may be able to do this in a high-powered blender using the tamper, but be sure to stop to scrape the sides and take breaks because it will be hard on the motor. Don't overmix here - you want the dates to be slightly chunky and not completely incorporated.

3. Transfer the mixture to the spring-form pan and spread evenly along the bottom with a spatula.

4. Bake in the oven for 18-20 minutes, or until a knife comes out clean when gently inserted. Set aside to cool.

5. Combine all of the filling ingredients, cold in a pot.

6. Turn the heat on medium-low, and heat, stirring constantly, for 5-10 minutes. The mixture should liquefy and the gelatin should dissolve.

7. If you still have some chunks after 10 minutes, transfer to a blender and blend for a few seconds to incorporate.

8. Pour into the spring-form pan over the gingersnap crust.

9. Place in the refrigerator to set for at least 3 hours.

10. To make the frosting, combine all of the ingredients in a small bowl. A thick, spreadable frosting should form. If it is too runny, add more arrowroot, a teaspoon at a time until desired thickness is reached. The frosting will harden when placed in the refrigerator and soften at room temperature (although it shouldn't melt).

11. When you are ready to frost your cake, you can either use a frosting kit or apply it to the top with a spatula.

Summer Pasta(less) Salad

Preparation time

50 minutes

Ingredients

- 2 1/2 lb Yellow Squash, peeled and spiralized into noodles

- 1/2 cup Green Onion, sliced

- 1/2 whole Cucumber, quartered and sliced

- 6 oz Black Olives

- 1/2 cup Olive Oil, Extra Virgin, (for the dressing)

- 3 Tbsp Apple Cider Vinegar, (for the dressing)

- 1/2 tsp Garlic Powder, (for the dressing)

- 3/4 tsp Onion Powder, (for the dressing)

- 1 1/2 tsp Oregano, dried, (for the dressing)

- (caution: the strictest form of AIP eliminates black pepper, leave it out if you are sensitive)NaN

- 1/8 tsp Thyme, (for the dressing)

- 1/2 tsp Basil, dried, (for the dressing)

- 3/4 tsp Parsley, (for the dressing)

- 3/4 tsp Sea Salt, (for the dressing)

Instructions

1. Place all veggies in a large bowl.

2. Place all dressing ingredients in a small glass jar. Shake in mix thoroughly.

3. Pour dressing over veggies and toss to combine.

4. Serve cold.

Strawberry, Rose, and Coconut Milkshake

Preparation time

10 minutes

Ingredients

• 2 cup Coconut Meat, freshly scooped from a Young Thai Coconut

- 2 1/4 cup Coconut Water, freshly poured from a Young Thai Coconut

- 1 cup Strawberries, fresh or frozen

- 1 Tbsp Rose Water, food grade

- 1/2 cup Ice Cubes, optional-use only if using fresh strawberries

- 1 whole Coconut Cream, optional-for topping

Instructions

1. Whip the coconut cream in a large bowl using a hand or stand mixer, until fluffy. Set aside.

2. Place the coconut meat and coconut water in a high powered blender, and blend on high, until smooth and creamy.

3. Add the frozen strawberries and rose water, and continue to blend until there are no lumps.

4. Pour the milkshake into glasses, top with the whipped coconut cream, and serve.

Hydrating Berry Popsicles

Preparation time

12 hours

Ingredients

- 1 1/2 cups Blackberries

- 1 1/2 cups Blueberries

- 3 cups Strawberries

- 3 cups Coconut Water, unsweetened

- 2 Tbsp Honey, Raw

Instructions

1. Place the blackberries, one cup of coconut water, and two teaspoons of honey into a blender. Blend until smooth.

2. Strain the mixture through a fine mesh strainer to remove the blackberry seeds, and set aside.

3. Repeat this process two more times with the strawberries and blueberries, using 1 cup of coconut water per flavor of berry, and 2 teaspoons of honey.

4. Be sure that all three flavors are strained into separate bowls.

5. Pour the blueberries in the first 3rd of your popsicle molds, and freeze until solid.

6. Repeat with the strawberries and blackberries.

7. Once you have filled the last flavor into your molds, freeze overnight, or for at least 6 hours.

Tempura Shrimp

Preparation time

1 hour 10 minutes

Ingredients

- 3/4 cup Arrowroot Flour

- 1/4 cup Cassava Flour, plus 2 tablespoons

- 2 tsp Baking Powder

- 1/8 tsp Ginger, ground

- 1/2 tsp Himalayan Pink Salt

- 1/8 tsp Fish Sauce, about 3 drops

- 1 cup Sparkling Water

- 2 Tbsp Coconut Aminos

- Coconut Oil, Organic, Tropical Traditions steam refined coconut oil. Aim for at least 2 inches of oil in pot

- 2 lb Shrimp, Raw, wild caught, tail on

Instructions

1. Whisk together the dry ingredients in a large mixing bowl; only adding the 1/4 of cassava to start.

2. Pour in the fish sauce, coconut aminos, and sparkling water while whisking to combine. If batter is too loose, add a tablespoon of cassava at a time until the batter is about as thick as pancake batter (it should coat the whisk).

3. Choose a pot with high walls and a small diameter to maximize oil depth for frying. Add enough coconut oil (or lard, or your choice of cooking fat) to have a minimum depth of 3" of oil. Heat to 320 degrees Fahrenheit, monitoring the temperature with a candy thermometer.

4. Clean and peel the shrimp, removing all shell and only leaving the tail on. De-vein the shrimp.

5. Prepare a wire rack over a cookie sheet to allow fried shrimp to drain.

6. Dip the shrimp in the batter to coat, one at a time. Slowly lower into the hot oil, holding the shrimp by the tail, and allowing the batter to being to fry before releasing the shrimp. This will prevent the shrimp from sticking to the pot.

7. Working with only 2-3 shrimp in the pot at a time, cook the shrimp for about 3 minutes, until the batter is golden brown. Place on a wire rack to drain. Repeat until all shrimp are fried.

Blackberry Cobbler

Preparation time

50 minutes

Ingredients

• 12 oz Blackberries

• 2 Tbsp Coconut Oil, Organic, plus more for greasing

• 3 Tbsp Water

• 1/4 cup Arrowroot Flour

• 1/4 cup Coconut Flour

• 1/4 cup Honey, Raw

- 1/4 tsp Salt

- 3/4 tsp Baking Soda

- 1 1/4 tsp Lemon Juice

Instructions

1. Preheat oven to 300. Lightly grease an 8×8 baking dish with coconut oil.

2. Spread blackberries evenly in bottom of pan.

3. Mix remaining ingredients on medium speed until combined. Spread over blackberries.

4. Bake for 35-40 minutes, until entire top is golden brown.

Beets and Sweets Hash

Preparation time

55 minutes

Ingredients

- 1 whole Sweet Potato, peeled and cubed to 1/4" pieces

- 1 whole Beets, peeled and cubed to 1/4" pieces

- 2 Tbsp Olive Oil, Extra Virgin

- 3 pieces Bacon, chopped

- 2 whole Green Onion, chopped

Instructions

1. preheat oven to 375F

2. coat potato and beet cubes with olive oil, salt and pepper

3. roast for 35-40 minutes until fork tender

4. dice bacon and cook until crispy, drain fat reserving 1T

5. add beets and sweets to the pan and heat together with bacon and reserved bacon fat

6. garnish with chopped scallions and serve

Orange Teriyaki Meatballs

Preparation time

45 minutes

Ingredients

- 2 lb Chicken Breasts, boneless skinless, Ground

- 1/2 cup Green Onion, chopped

- 2 Tbsp Orange Zest

- 2/3 cup Orange Juice, fresh

- 2 tsp Ginger Root, minced

- 1/4 cup Coconut Aminos

- 1 Tbsp Apple Cider Vinegar

- 1 clove Garlic, minced

- 1 Tbsp Honey, Raw

Instructions

1. In a bowl, mix ground chicken (you can use any kind; breast or a blend) orange zest, pinch salt and green onions. On a parchment lined cookie sheet, form 2 1/2 inch sized meatballs.

2. Bake at 350 until internal temperature reaches 170 degrees. Mine took about 30 minutes.

3. In a saucepan, add coconut aminos grated ginger, garlic, honey, vinegar and fresh orange juice.

4. Bring to a simmer and reduce until sauce coats the back of a spoon. It will simmer for about 10 minutes and then start to watch it closely. It will start to foam and bubble as it is reducing and almost ready. You want the sauce to be the consistency of maple syrup.

5. When meatballs are cooked, place in a bowl and drizzle with the sauce. Gently toss to coat all the meatballs.

Warm Shrimp Salad with Bok Choy

Preparation time

15 minutes

Ingredients

- 1 head Bok Choy, large

- 1/3 lb Shrimp, Raw

- 1/4 tsp Fish Sauce

- 3 Tbsp Coconut Aminos

- 2 clove Garlic

- 1/4 cup Watercress

Instructions

1. Heat a large skillet over medium-high heat.

2. Rinse the bok choy, and remove the large white veins near the bottom of each leaf. Chop the leaves lengthwise, and set aside.

3. Place the shrimp in the skillet, and stir in the fish sauce and coconut aminos. Sauté for 4-5 minutes.

4. Add the minced garlic and watercress, and continue to sauté until the shrimp is completely opaque.

5. Add the bok choy, and sauté 1-2 minutes, until it begins to soften slightly.

6. Remove the skillet from the heat, and serve immediately.

Turkey Breakfast Sausage

Preparation time

12 minutes

Ingredients

- 1 lb Ground Turkey

- 1 Tbsp Primal Palate Breakfast Blend

- 1/2 Tbsp Lard

Instructions

1. Mix the ground turkey and spice blend in a bowl thoroughly. Form into patties by dividing

the mixture in half, then in half again, and all portions in half one last time (giving you 8 small patties).

2. Heat the lard, or you choice of cooking fat, over medium heat in a skillet. Fry the patties about 4-5 minutes on each side, until fully cooked (may take 10 minutes, or longer, depending on the thickness.)

3. Serve alongside your favorite breakfast dishes!

Slow Cooker Ham

Preparation time

5 hours

Ingredients

- 4 - 6 lb Ham

- 1/4 cup Honey, Raw

- 1/2 cup Orange Juice

- 2 tsp Rosemary, dried

- 4 Tbsp Coconut Oil, Organic

- 1 tsp Orange Zest

- 1 Tbsp Apple Cider Vinegar

Instructions

1. Place ham in slow cooker.

2. Put the rest of the ingredients on the ham.

3. Cook on low for 4-6 hours.

Sea Salt & Lime Spinach Chips

Preparation time

35 minutes

Ingredients

- 1 whole Lime, about 1 1/2 Tablespoons zest + 2 tsp juice, divided

- 1/2 tsp Sea Salt

- 8 cup Spinach, whole leaves, measured packed

- 2 Tbsp Olive Oil, Extra Virgin

Instructions

1. Preheat the oven to 275F. Line 2 baking sheets with nonstick pads, or lightly grease them.

2. In a small bowl, use your fingers to rub together the zest and the salt.

3. In a large mixing bowl, toss the spinach with the olive oil to thoroughly coat. Then add the lime salt and toss again to distribute a little bit of the salt on each leaf. Use your hands if necessary.

4. Distribute the spinach between the two prepared cookie sheets in an even layer (do not crowd the leaves). Sprinkle each batch with a teaspoon of lime juice.

5. Bake for 30-35 minutes (you may need less time depending on how fresh your spinach is, so keep an eye on it) until the leaves are withered and very thin.

6. Remove from oven, and let the chips cool completely on the pan before serving.

Breadsticks

Preparation time

20 minutes

Ingredients

- 4 Tbsp Olive Oil, Extra Virgin, divided (3 Tbsp for breadsticks, 1 Tbsp for topping)

- 3 Tbsp Water

- 1/3 cup Arrowroot Flour

- 1/3 cup Coconut Flour

- 1/2 tsp Baking Soda

- 1 tsp Rosemary, dried

- 1 1/2 tsp Lemon Juice

- 1 Tbsp Unflavored Gelatin, Beef, Great Lakes brand, plus 3 TBSP water (to create egg substitute)

- 1/8 tsp Garlic Powder, for topping

- 1/8 tsp Sea Salt, for topping

Instructions

1. Preheat oven to 350.

2. In standing mixer, place all ingredients except for gelatin egg substitute.

3. Prepare gelatin egg: Mix 1 tablespoon gelatin into 1 tablespoon cool water. Add 2 tablespoons of boiling water and whisk vigorously until completely dissolved and frothy. Add to mixing

bowl and combine on medium until a thick dough forms.

4. Scrape dough onto sheet of parchment paper. Divide dough into 8 balls. Grease hands with olive oil and roll each ball into 8" sticks. If dough cracks, wet your fingertips to add a bit more moisture.

5. Brush breadsticks evenly with olive oil. Sprinkle garlic and sea salt over top.

6. Bake 10-12 minutes, until tops are golden brown.

Starch-Free Coconut Cream Pie

Preparation time

45 minutes

Ingredients

* 1/2 cup Coconut Flour, (for the crust)

* 1/4 tsp Salt, (for the crust)

* 1/4 tsp Baking Soda, (for the crust)

* 3/4 tsp Cinnamon, ground, (for the crust)

* 1/3 cup Coconut Oil, Organic, melted (for the crust)

* 1/2 tsp Pure Vanilla Extract, (for the crust)

- 1/3 cup Honey, Raw, (for the filling)

- 2 tsp Gelatin, Unflavored, Knox brand, (for the filling)

- 1 cup Coconut, shredded, toasted at 350 for 5-6 minutes (for the filling)

- 16 oz Coconut Milk, (for the filling)

- 1/2 cup Coconut Butter, Organic, (for the filling)

- 1 1/2 tsp Vanilla Extract, (for the filling)

- 1/4 tsp Sea Salt, (for the filling)

Instructions

1. For the crust

2. Preheat oven to 350.

3. In small bowl, whisk together dry ingredients: coconut flour, salt, baking soda and cinnamon. Set aside.

4. In stand mixer, beat wet ingredients together on medium.

5. Add dry ingredients, mixing until fully combined.

6. Scrape dough into 9" pie plate. Place a piece of parchment paper (large enough to cover entire pie plate) over the crust. Using small hand-held rolling pin (or use a small drinking glass turned on its side), roll crust flat to cover the bottom and sides of the pie plate. The dough will thicken as the gelatin sets, so this may take some extra rolling compared to an egg-based crust.

7. Bake for 10-12 minutes, until golden brown. While crust is baking, toast coconut and prepare pie filling.

For the filling

1. Toast coconut on a baking sheet for 5-6 minutes, until golden brown (Do not skip this step. Without it, the pie will be colorless and semi-translucent. It also adds great toasty flavor!)

2. In medium saucepan over medium heat, Whisk all ingredients together, except for the gelatin and toasted coconut.

3. Scoop out 2 teaspoons of the milk mixture and place it into a small dish. Add the gelatin

and let it absorb the milk to create a rubbery mixture.

4. Cover the milk mixture and bring to a simmer. Whisk in rubbery gelatin mixture and whisk vigorously until the gelatin is completely dissolved. Turn off heat.

5. Stir in the coconut, and pour the mixture into the prepared graham pie crust.

6. Refrigerate for 4 hours, until completely cool and hardened throughout.

Maple Brown Sugar N'Oatmeal

Preparation time

15 minutes

Ingredients

* 1 head Cauliflower, broken into 1-inch florets

* 4 Tbsp Coconut Oil, Organic, divided

* 3 Tbsp Coconut Milk

* 2 Tbsp Coconut Palm Sugar

* 2 Tbsp Maple Syrup, Pure, plus more for drizzling (optional)

- 1/4 tsp Sea Salt, heaping

- 1/4 tsp Cinnamon, ground, plus more for sprinkling (optional)

- 1 pinch Cloves, ground

Instructions

1. Preheat the oven to 425 degrees F. Line a large baking sheet with foil.

2. In a large, microwave-safe bowl, heat 2 tablespoons of coconut oil in the microwave until it's melted. Add the cauliflower florets and drizzle over 2 tablespoons of melted coconut oil. Toss the cauliflower florets and toss with your hands or a large spoon until the cauliflower is completely coated with oil.

3. Lay the florets in a single, even layer on the baking sheet. Place the baking sheet in the oven and roast the cauliflower for 20-25 minutes or until tender and the edges are turning a deep brown.

4. Remove the baking sheet from the oven and add the roasted cauliflower, 2 tablespoons coconut oil, coconut milk, sugar, maple syrup, salt, cinnamon, and cloves to the bowl of a large food processor. Process on high for 3 minutes, or until the mixture is thick, creamy, and blended.

5. Spoon into bowls, top with cinnamon and maple syrup and/or fresh fruit (optional) and enjoy!

Festive Green Spritzer

Preparation time

5 minutes

Ingredients

- 1 whole Cucumber, medium

- 1 whole Lemon, large

- 3 whole Pear, Bartlett

- 3 whole Kale, large leaves

- 1 oz Ginger Root, three inch piece

- 16 oz Sparkling Water

Instructions

1. Peel some of the rind off the lemon and core the pears.

2. Put the cucumber, lemon, pears, kale, and ginger through the juicer.

3. Pour the mixture through a fine mesh sieve. Fill a tall glass with ice and add about one cup of juice concentrate.

4. Top with about u00bd cup of club soda and enjoy! Adjust club soda and juice to taste.

Cauliflower Rice

Preparation time

20 minutes

Ingredients

- 1 clove Garlic, minced

- 1 Tbsp Coconut Oil, Organic

- 1 head Cauliflower

- 1/2 cup Yellow Onion, chopped

- 1/2 tsp Himalayan Pink Salt, to taste (and black pepper, if not following AIP)

- 1 tsp Primal Palate Garlic & Herb Seasoning, (sub: 1/2 tsp himalayan pink salt)

Instructions

1. Rinse cauliflower under cool water and pat dry.

2. Using a cheese grater, grate the cauliflower to a coarse texture (approximately the size of rice grains). Using a food processor to pulse the cauliflower to desired texture works as well.

3. Heat the coconut oil in a skillet over medium heat.

4. Sauté the onion and garlic for 3–4 minutes, or until the onion is relatively translucent.

5. Add in the cauliflower rice and continue to sauté for 4–5 minutes.

6. Season with salt and pepper, and serve.

Carob Chip Bars

Preparation time

50 minutes

Ingredients

* 2 whole Plantain, peeled and chopped

* 1/2 cup Pumpkin Puree

* 2 Tbsp Tigernut Flour

* 1/2 tsp Baking Soda

* 3 Tbsp Coconut Butter, Organic

* 1/4 cup Coconut Oil, Organic

* 2 Tbsp Honey, Raw

- 2 cup Coconut Milk, chilled, just the cream

Instructions

1. preheat oven to 350 deg

2. place all ingredients in bowl of food processor and blend until smooth, a couple minutes

3. pour into a greased loaf pan

4. stir in 1/2 c carob chips by hand

5. bake for 40-50 min (until inserted knife comes out clean)

6. meanwhile, whip coconut cream (i used my food processor)

7. once bars are done, cool on counter the in the fridge for a couple hours

8. frost with whip cream and rechill in fridge

One Pot Steamed Garlic and Herb Scallops with Veggies

Preparation time

15 minutes

Ingredients

- 1/3 cup Water, or broth

- 1 Tbsp Olive Oil, Extra Virgin

- 1 Tbsp Lemon Juice

- 1 pinch Sea Salt

- 1/4 tsp Basil, dried

- 1/4 tsp Onion Powder, or onion salt

- 1/4 tsp Garlic, minced

- 6 oz Scallops, 1 serving (4-5 medium to large)

- 1 cup Kale, spinach, greens or favorite vegetables - chopped

- 2 Tbsp Greek Salad Dressing (click for recipe) , Dressing of choice.

Instructions

1. Place water and dash salt in small pot. Place steamer on top. In a separate bowl, toss your scallops in a bit of your favorite dressing (maybe 1-2 tbsp) and then add in your seasoning. Boil your water then Place scallops and veggies on

top of steamer. cover and steam with boiled water for 7-8 minutes or until scallops are opaque.

2. Remove from pot and place everything on plate. Add more seasoning and dash of lemon juice.

3. Scallops serve one but you can add more and make it serve two or more!

4. Check scallops and veggies around 7-8 minutes to see if they are done.

5. Scallops are done when they are opaque in center and easy to slice, not chewy. You really can't undercook them.

6. If you are using smaller scallops, they will probably cook faster, around 5-6 minutes steamed.

Miso Glazed Salmon

Preparation time

30 minutes

Ingredients

• 16 oz Salmon Filet, Wild Caught, 4 (4 ounce filets)

• 1 Tbsp Maple Syrup, Pure

• 2 Tbsp Coconut Aminos

• 2 Tbsp Water, warm

Instructions

1. Preheat oven to 350 degrees

2. Add all ingredients except salmon to a sauce pan

3. Heat over medium heat, stirring frequently, until glaze is formed (5-7 minutes)

4. Place salmon filets on baking sheet lined with parchment paper

5. brush glaze onto fish

6. bake for 20 minutes or until fish flakes easily with a fork, pausing to reglaze every 5 minutes

7. garnish with green onions and sesame seeds

Bison Stew

Preparation time

6 hours 20 minutes

Ingredients

- 2 lb Bison Steak Medallions

- 1 Tbsp Coconut Oil, Organic

- 2 cup Celery, chopped

- 3 sprig Thyme

- 3 sprig Rosemary, fresh

- 1 head Cauliflower, chopped

- 1 Yellow Onion, chopped

- 1 quart Beef Broth, reduced sodium

- 1/2 tsp Salt, to taste (and black pepper, if not following AIP)

Instructions

1. In a cast iron skillet, brown bison stew meat on all sides in coconut oil.

2. Transfer seared bison meat into a large soup pot.

3. Place chopped onion and celery into the pot with the bison.

4. Pour beef broth over meat.

5. Season liberally with salt and pepper.

6. Place herbs, and celery greens into the pot, and turn burner onto medium heat.

7. Bring stew to a boil, stirring often.

8. Once stew comes to a boil, turn heat down to low, and cover with a lid.

9. Simmer stew for 6-8 hours, adding the chopped cauliflower for the last hour of cooking.

Roasted Rosemary Beets

Preparation time

15 minutes

Ingredients

- 2 Tbsp Olive Oil, Extra Virgin

- 2 Tbsp Rosemary, fresh, chopped

- 3 Beets, chopped

- 1/2 tsp Salt, (and black pepper, if not following AIP)

Instructions

1. Preheat the oven to roast at 400°F.

2. In a baking dish, toss beets in olive oil, salt, pepper, and rosemary.

3. Roast beets for 35 minutes, or until crispy on the outside and tender in the center.

Sweet + Tangy Pork Lettuce Wraps

Preparation time

35 minutes

Ingredients

- 1 head Lettuce, Iceburg

- 1 whole Carrots, Small size head

- 1/4 head Red Cabbage, Small size head

- 1 whole Mango, Sliced

- 1/4 cup Mint Leaves, Chopped

- 1/4 cup Cilantro, Chopped

- 1/2 whole Red Onion, Chopped

- 1 pieces Ginger Root, 1 inch piece

- 1 clove Garlic, Finely chopped

- 2 Tbsp Red Wine Vinegar

- 3 Tbsp Honey, Raw

- 4 Tbsp Coconut Aminos

- 1/8 tsp Sea Salt

- 1 Tbsp Olive Oil, Extra Virgin

- 1 Tbsp Orange Juice

- 1 lb Ground Pork

Instructions

1. Wash iceberg lettuce and cut into quarters. Peel leaves off to create wraps. Set aside.

2. Wash mango and cut into cubes.

3. Peel and chop red onion. Set aside.

4. Peel and julienne or thinly slice carrot and set aside.

5. Wash and chop mint and set aside.

6. Wash and chop cilantro and set aside.

7. Peel and finely chop ginger and garlic clove and set aside.

8. In a separate bowl add honey and warm just until it becomes a liquid. Add vinegar, coconut aminos, sea salt, ginger, garlic and orange juice. Mix well to combine. Set sauce aside.

9. In a skillet add olive oil and meat. Break up meat and stir continually until it is half cooked. This should take about 5-10 min.

10. Add onions and cook an additional 5 min. Stir every minute or so.

11. Add sauce, mix well and cook another 5-10 min or until meat is browned and sauce starts to thicken. Stir every few minutes.

12. To serve place a spoonful of pork on top of a lettuce leaf and top with cabbage, carrot, cilantro, mint and mango.

AIP Pizzette

Preparation time

50 minutes

Ingredients

- 1/3 cup Coconut Flour, (crust)

- 1/3 cup Arrowroot Powder, (crust)

- 1/3 cup Tapioca Starch, (crust)

- 1 Tbsp Unflavored Gelatin, Beef, Great Lakes brand, (crust)

- 6 Tbsp Lard, (crust) at room temperature, soft but not melted

- 1/2 cup Water, (crust)

- 1 tsp Salt, (crust)

- 1/4 lb Pepperoni, Uncured, (filling)

- 2 Tbsp Basil, fresh, (filling) chopped

- 1 cup Caulifredo Sauce (click for recipe)

- Buy on Amazon

Instructions

1. [For the crust] Mix together dry ingredients (coconut, tapioca and arrowroot flours, gelatin, and salt).

2. Blend in lard using a fork or pastry blender.

3. Mix water in, stirring until a ball of dough forms.

4. Wet your hands, then place the ball of dough on a parchment-lined pizza stone.

5. Flatten the dough with your palms, then place another sheet of parchment over the top.

6. Using a rolling pin, flatten the dough into a big circle.

7. Roll out to about 1/4" thickness. You can use your hand to run a little more water around the edges if it threatens to crack.

8. Remove top parchment and prepare the fillings.

9. [For the filling] Spread sauce over crust, leaving 2-3 inches bare on edges.

10. Top with meat, basil and any additional toppings of choice.

11. Using the parchment paper underneath, carefully fold up the edges of the crust over the edge of the fillings, again spreading a little water over the crust if need be.

12. Cook at 425 for 25 minutes.

Bacon-wrapped Shrimp

Preparation time

50 minutes

Ingredients

1. 1 1/2 lb Shrimp, Raw, and tail-on

2. 18 oz Bacon

3. Instructions

4. Cut the strips of bacon in half. Wrap each shrimp, starting from the head and working toward the tail. Skewer each shrimp with a 4-inch toothpick.

5. Preheat your oven to 350 degrees Fahrenheit. Place the skewered shrimp on a parchment-lined, rimmed baking sheet. Cook for 30 minutes, or until the bacon is crisp and the shrimp is cooked through (opaque).